Emotional Eating
with Diabetes

Your guide to creating a positive relationship with food.

Ginger Vieira • Wellness & Diabetes Coach
Foreword by William Polonsky PhD, CDE

Living in Progress Publishing

DISCLAIMER

This book is not intended as a substitute for the medical recommendations of physicians or other health care providers. The information in this book is intended to help the readers cooperate with physicians and health care professionals in a joint quest for optimum health and wellness. Neither the publisher nor the author is responsible for any goods and/or services referred to in this book.

First printing December 2012
First edition

ISBN 978-0-9884523-0-5

Photography by Chris Valites, chrisvalites.com
Interior and Exterior design by Jessica Piccirilli

FOR MY MOTHER,

who fed us so many vegetables with dinner
and kept plenty of candy in the "candy drawer."

CONTENTS

Foreword by William Polonsky PhD, CDE   1

1. Emotional Eating with Diabetes   3

2. Habits that Lead to Overeating   8

3. Over-treating Low Blood Sugars   14

4. Using Food to Hide Your Emotions   19

5. A Positive Relationship with Food   28

6. Setting Yourself Up for Success   36

7. You Are Living in Progress   41

Resources & Support   43

FOREWORD

It is a crazy world we live in, and diabetes just makes it all a bit crazier. And as we all know so well, one of those crazy-making issues is food. For all Americans, and especially for American women, there is unrelenting pressure to "watch your weight" and to eat as healthfully as possible. At the same time, of course, our media and culture bombard us with temptations that lead us in the opposite direction.

It is perhaps then no surprise that so many of us end up at war with food: it is the enemy, yet it is also what gives us comfort and pleasure. We must not ever surrender, and yet we must. As a diabetes psychologist, I recognize that this war is often magnified when people are living with diabetes. More than 25 years ago, when I saw my first patient with diabetes, our discussion centered on the emotional battle over food. And just yesterday, the last patient I saw — yes, we were talking about food. Popular subject, no?

Scientific research has shown us that eating problems and more serious eating disorders are more likely to occur when an individual is inundated with rules and constraints about what to eat. The more we are told to limit ourselves, to control ourselves, the more often there is an impulse to leap free from those shackles. But the resulting eating binge is not necessarily so fun; it is typically accompanied—sooner or later-- by feelings of shame, guilt, anger, frustration, sadness and so much more. And when you develop a condition like diabetes, where suddenly there seem to be some many rules and constraints regarding what you should and shouldn't eat (even though most of those rules are completely unnecessary and not relevant to the way diabetes is treated in the 21st century), the risk for developing an unhealthy relationship with food is much more likely.

Bottom line: If you are living with diabetes and struggling around issues with food, this is completely understandable. You are not a bad person, and you are not alone.

One of the key solutions is to realize that you can never be perfect with your diabetes nor can you be perfect when it comes to following a diabetes-friendly way of eating. And you don't need to be. There is no need for guilt or shame; you've done nothing wrong. Though it isn't easy, what is needed is an armistice: it is time to make peace with food. In this book, Ginger Viera does a lovely job of explaining and addressing the problem of emotional eating in diabetes. She cuts through the professional gobbledygook (the unnecessary jargon which we psychologists are too prone to use), and cuts to the heart of issue. And she does it with real heart, too. Are you ready start feeling better? Fasten your seat belt and get ready for your adventure with Ginger!

William H. Polonsky PhD, CDE
Associate Clinical Professor, University of California, San Diego
CEO, Behavioral Diabetes Institute
BehavioralDiabetesInstitute.org

1 Emotional Eating with Diabetes

In life with diabetes, food is never just food. We cannot simply sit down at the dinner table and begin to eat. Instead, every meal and snack, even a small glass of milk or juice, has consequences if we don't put diabetes first.

At breakfast, lunch, and dinner, we work. And we hope that the insulin and medications we took for the carbohydrates we counted (or guessed) was accurate. We work so hard to do a job every day that our bodies are supposed to do on their own: produce and use insulin to manage our blood sugar levels around food, exercise, stress, and so much more. But with diabetes, that becomes our job instead. And it's never easy.

Inevitably, this begins to impact how we think about food. When we sit down to a meal, we look at the delicious food on our plates and a variety of thoughts quickly run through our minds:

- Should I be eating this?

- I have absolutely no idea how many carbs are in this meal...whatever, I don't care anymore. I'm just gonna take a big dose of insulin...see what happens.

- I probably should not be eating this.

- This is definitely, absolutely, totally going to screw up my blood sugar later today. I don't care. I'm used to it. That's just life with diabetes.

- I'm such a bad diabetic for eating this.

- I'm sick of carb-counting and taking shots.

- I'm supposed to eat the perfect diet.

- I can't be perfect. What's wrong with me?

And it doesn't stop there. Next, we get to press a few buttons on our insulin pumps, draw back several units of insulin in our insulin pens and syringes, or take several pills. Sure, that sounds easy enough. None of that could possibly take more than thirty seconds or so, at the most. Big deal, right?

Well, yes, it is a big deal, because we are going through that entire process every day, at every meal. And it isn't a perfect process either. If we over-guess or under-guess the amount of carbohydrates in that serving of potatoes, we'll be dealing with the consequences for the next several hours, battling high and low blood sugars. If we exercise before that meal, or after that meal, it completely changes how we take insulin for that meal.

If we're beyond stressed studying for exams, going through a divorce, in the process of buying a new house, or recovering from the loss of a loved one, then everything in our diabetes management is impacted, too. Those regular parts of life can completely change how much insulin our body needs for dinner, or the whole day. Maybe more insulin. Maybe less.

Did I mention that in life with diabetes, we are constantly being told what we should or should not be eating? What we can and we cannot be eating. While non-diabetics can eat food that none of us "ought" to be eating, the impact that food has on every human body isn't nearly as obvious unless you live with diabetes. Every casual treat or "mistake" stares back at you on your meter the next time you check your blood sugar.

Signs of Emotional Eating

- You eat very little all day, and too much at night.

- You turn to food so you can avoid feeling your emotions: fear, stress, anger, sadness, loneliness, guilt, and pain.

- Your behavior around food leaves you feeling guilty and ashamed of yourself.

- You use food as a way to punish your body and spite your diabetes.

- You eat very differently in public than at home.

- You often tell yourself you have no will-power or self-control.

- Specific types of food seem to trigger an uncontrollable need to binge.

- You think about food constantly, and feel trapped by this part of your life.

- You regularly try to eliminate a type of food or entire food group in an attempt to gain control over your behavior around that food.

Like carbohydrates. Carbohydrates of any kind come with a double-edged sword. We're often told we shouldn't eat too many or sometimes any of certain kinds of carbohydrates.

Carbohydrates become a feared enemy. Something we struggle to balance our lives around. They require so much work, so much counting and adjusting for. One mistake in our measurement around carbohydrates can ruin the rest of our day.

Meanwhile, carbohydrates are the only thing that can literally save our lives.

We hide different forms of carbohydrates in every nook and cranny of our cars, our bags and purses, next to our beds, attached with a rubber band to the handlebars of our bicycles. And you'll know you're in a yoga class with me when there's a container of glucose tabs placed carefully at the top of my yoga mat.

We spend half our day feeling guilty we ate carbohydrates, and the other half of the day desperately trying to save our own lives with carbohydrates during a low blood sugar.

It's hardly surprising that the weight of living with this high-maintenance disease also comes with an insanely immense pressure to eat all the right foods at exactly the right times. That pressure can lead to a messy, confused, imbalanced relationship with food. The pressure around food isn't always easy to see, either.

Scott Johnson's Story

"I feel a lot of anger around food. I feel anger especially when I have to count and measure everything.

It feels like diabetes is controlling how much I can eat, and it really pisses me off.

Sometimes that anger triggers an episode of binge eating. The binge on food might feel good and seem like a way to regain a bit of that control. But when I'm miserably full with a high blood sugar I know I have only hurt myself. This leaves me feeling ashamed, guilty, and weak.

I haven't regained any control. Instead, I've done the exact opposite!

Eating with diabetes is so full of math and mechanics that I wonder if I can recognize the natural signals that are supposed to come with food. Feeling satisfied? What is that? How about a low blood sugar with a full stomach? How confusing (and frustrating)!

Diabetes has scrambled my relationship with food, and that makes me angry. I haven't resolved this yet, but I am making progress."

Counting carbohydrates and taking insulin might be what everyone else around us can see, and they usually say things like, "Oh, wow. I don't know how you do that every day." In their eyes, the injection of that dauntingly sharp needle is the hardest part.

In reality, the sharp needle is actually pretty easy. The pain of stabbing our bodies doesn't go away, but we eventually accept it as pain we'll experience every day. The hard part is living every single day with a disease that revolves around the food we eat, and the food we've been told we should not ever eat.

Your imbalanced relationship with food has developed gradually since your diagnosis. It continues to evolve every time someone tells you to avoid eating pizza, ice cream, fries, bread, chips, bagels, and candy. The list goes on and on.

In this book, we are going to untwist, unravel, and let go of your current relationship with food. We are going to build completely new ways of thinking about what you can eat, and the many foods you were once told you should never eat.

We are going to look closely at what drives you to use food as a weapon against yourself and against your diabetes.

Our final goal is to build a relationship with food that leaves you feeling proud of your choices, never deprived, and with the knowledge that you are giving your body and your life with diabetes the compassion that you need and deserve.

Cherise Shockley's Story

"For a person with diabetes, a cupcake is never just a cupcake; it's a flavorful, mathematical equation. We cannot easily walk up to the bakery for a cupcake and simply enjoy it.

After picking the flavor, we have to calculate the carbohydrates, insulin doses, and hope our estimated calculation works out well in the end. If we don't estimate perfectly, we can end up feeling incredibly guilty.

How do I shift my thinking from seeing a cupcake as a tedious, mathematical equation to actually

enjoying that cupcake without an overpowering feeling of guilt?

I remind myself of this:

Yes, I have diabetes, but I can and will treat myself to a cupcake from time to time while doing my best to manage my diabetes. I can choose a flavor. Estimate the carbohydrates. Take my insulin. And keep a close eye on my blood sugar afterwards in case my estimate wasn't perfect.

I deserve it, and so do you."

A **healthy** relationship with **food** is about **feeling proud** of your choices, whether you choose **carrots** or **ice cream**.

② Habits that Lead to Overeating

You may have tried many times to change your relationship with food. Maybe you've vowed to never binge on food again during a low blood sugar, to never eat a whole pint of ice cream after a stressful day, and maybe you've even promised to never eat another gram of carbohydrate (or at least another potato chip) ever again in your entire life.

And it didn't work. Within hours, days, or weeks you were back where you started.

You're not alone.

On our own, we tend to skip the very crucial step of acknowledging what's really going on in our life, in our habits, and most importantly, in our thoughts that leads to our self-destructive behavior with food.

We overlook the first step where we actually acknowledge what really needs to change. In this chapter, we're going to look at the three habits that commonly happen in the life of any person who struggles with overeating.

The first habit is the development of "rules" that you have set for yourself. We built these rules over time in an effort to gain control over our actions and emotions, but more often than not, they simply backfire.

The second is the simple habit of starving your metabolism during the day because you're trying to eat fewer and fewer calories. This inevitably leads to overeating.

The third habit is the mindset of your decision process, constantly telling yourself that you "can't eat this" and you "can't eat that." Instead, we're going to build a mindset that empowers, not limits.

Let's take a deeper look at these habits:

"Rules" around food that do more harm than good:

- I shouldn't eat carbohydrates whatsoever.
- I shouldn't eat late at night.
- I'm not going to eat any _____ anymore, ever again!
- If I eat any _____ then that means I've screwed up entirely!
- I should try to eat as little as possible all day long.
- I should try to avoid _____ because I love it too much.
- Eating any sweets, treats, or junk food that I love is bad.
- Fats are bad.
- Carbohydrates are bad.
- Meat, cheese, and peanut butter are bad.
- All food is bad.

The trouble with these "rules" is that they give food more and more power over us. The more we try to restrain ourselves from a certain food, the more we binge on it when another part of our life feels out of our control, or simply when we're hungry.

These rules also leave very few choices and require total, absolute perfection. I don't know about you, but I cannot be perfect. Good news: we don't need to be perfect in order to be healthy.

Instead, we can plan our sweets and treats. We will expect "mistakes" and imperfections in our overall nutrition plan. No food is "bad." All food is just food. These changes in your "rules" around what you eat are crucial. You'll look deeper into this part of your life in Chapter 5.

Diabetes First. Dessert Second.

Diabetes management is absolutely our first priority when it comes to how we eat. But if depriving ourselves leads to overeating and high blood sugars, then learning how to include treats, in moderation, with proper insulin doses and our prescribed medications is the secret.

When I include a treat in my diet, I count the carbohdyrates carefully and take an accurate amount of insulin. I also plan my treats only when and if my blood sugar is in a healthy range, and checking my blood sugar often after the treat

If you're not on insulin, then you can find room in your diet for a treat in two ways: swapping it for another form of carbohydrate you usually eat, or choosing a treat like an expensive cheese or bacon to enjoy instead, which won't raise your blood sugar.

The end goal is still the same: you're giving yourself the freedom to be imperfect and enjoy a special treat. Think about the best treat for your diabetes, and the smartest way to make room in your day for that treat.

Are you starving your metabolism?

Instead of thinking of food as something you want to avoid, eventually you can think of it as something you enjoy that also feeds you, fuels you, and keeps you healthy.

Many people who binge on food at night have starved themselves during the day. Your body needs calories, and it will demand that you eat those calories all at once, late at night, if it has to. Starve yourself during the day = overeat at night.

Think of your metabolism like a burning fire: if you stop adding wood to the fire, the flame will die down and eventually go out. When you don't eat enough calories during the day, consuming just a few or none between breakfast and dinner, your metabolism actually thinks you're starving it. Purposely.

It says, "Well, Alex isn't feeding me, so I might as well slow down, and burn as little body fat as I can." This applies to skipping breakfast, too. By not eating often enough you are actually telling your metabolism to burn less—to conserve energy, body fat, and calories. When you finally do feed your metabolism, it says, "Oh! Finally! I'm going to hold on to these calories as long as I can!"

Instead, when you eat small meals, often (every 3 to 4 hours), you are giving your metabolism a reason to burn! To fire up! To work hard! To use fat and calories. The easiest step to preventing overeating is to learn how to properly feed yourself throughout the day.

You will learn how to feed your metabolism in Chapter 5.

Crash Dieting 101

The term "crash-dieting" or "yo-yo dieting" implies that a person is constantly choosing strict diet plans for quick results. A crash-diet inevitably leads to failure because the plan is too strict and too difficult to maintain for very long.

If you choose a diet regimen or fad that you intentionally plan to follow for a short period of time for quick results, keep these points in mind:

- You are more likely to gain the weight back quickly because your severe diet can hinder your

metabolism, and you'll bounce back to old habits immediately afterwards.

- Crash-dieting becomes a self-destructive cycle because you're bound to fail if it's too strict to maintain for long. You'll revert to binge eating, and old habits, gain the weight back, and feel very guilty. The overall impact of this cycle on your self-esteem can be tremendous.

- Learning how to eat a balanced diet, with treats, is the key to ending your yo-yo dieting habits.

"I can't eat this" vs. "I choose to eat this"

In diabetes, we are trained by books, television, doctors, parents, and friends that we can not eat certain foods. We cannot eat candy, birthday cakes, ice cream, pizza, and chips. If it's delicious or fun, we probably can't (or shouldn't) eat it.

This is a quiet but significant conversation you have with yourself over and over, perhaps before every single meal you eat. And it doesn't help you. Instead, it might be making you feel as though the disease is trying to control you, limit you, and deprive you. You want to fight it. Gain control. Gain power over the disease by saying, "Shut up! I'm gonna eat whatever I want."

But you pay the price in guilt, denial, high blood sugars, and weight-gain. You abuse and overeat the food simply because it is "off-limits." In the end, your actions are still being controlled by food.

Imagine, instead, if you told yourself, "I can actually eat whatever I want. This is my body. I choose. I'm the one who puts the food in my mouth. No one can stop me."

Instead of feeling limited, you have every option, and every choice. You choose to respect your body by not overeating. Even when you choose candy, you are in control, not fighting. Instead of choosing candy with shame, in an attempt to fight against the reality of your life with diabetes, you are choosing it proudly, with awareness of your diabetes management. You take your insulin, and enjoy the food.

In Chapter 5, you will create this empowering mindset.

Choosing to Respect My Body

When I was diagnosed with celiac disease (an intolerance to gluten in bread, cakes, pizza, crackers, etc.) in the 8th grade, I couldn't help but think, "I'm not supposed to eat that bread; therefore, I want to eat it."

Even foods I'd never really liked before become irresistible. Like bagels, toast, and pizza. But when I told myself I "can't" eat those things, I only wanted them more. I saw them as something forbidden, something resembling a disease I didn't ask for, and wished I didn't have.

Eventually, I realized I can actually eat as much gluten as I want. Literally, I can grab it, put it in my mouth, and eat it. No one can stop me. I can eat whatever I want to eat. This is my body. I can hurt my body if I want to.

But I can choose not to. I can choose to say no, and choose things that are good for my body.

I find power in choosing to respect my body, instead of choosing to fight against the reality of my life with celiac.

What rules have you created around food? Do these rules harm you or help you?

_____

_____

_____

_____

_____

_____

Are you starving your metabolism during the day and overeating at night?

_____

_____

_____

_____

_____

_____

What foods do you overeat because you've labeled them as "forbidden"?

_____

_____

_____

_____

_____

_____

If you want to
eat candy,
say to yourself,
"I'm **choosing** to
eat this candy.
I'll take my **insulin,**
and **enjoy**
this candy."

③ Over-treating Low Blood Sugars

Overeating and emotional eating certainly aren't habits that exist only in people living with diabetes. Over-treating your low blood sugars, however, is a challenging habit that is unique to a life with diabetes.

Fact: the human brain relies on a second-by-second delivery of glucose (sugar) in order to function properly, to think, to wonder, to know the difference between red and blue. This fact helps explain why, during a low blood sugar, we can feel as though no amount of food will ever possibly be enough.

Binge-eating during a low blood sugar is common. It's easy to do because your brain keeps telling you: "More. More. More."

Worst of all, it will absolutely lead to further guilt and shame because overeating during that low blood sugar inevitably leads to weight gain, and an eventual high blood sugar.

The high blood sugar leads to guilt, and a required correction dose of insulin. And the glucose from that high blood sugar will eventually be stored as body fat, which leads to further weight gained from over-treating that low blood sugar.

This is a roller-coaster that feels impossible to get off of, but in the end, you do have a choice in how you treat your low blood sugars. But you do have the ability to prevent that roller-coaster from taking over the rest of your life around food. Does that mean the roller-coaster will never happen again? No, there are certainly variables in life with diabetes that are impossible to control, but you control the simplest variable: how you treat your low blood sugars.

In this chapter, you'll identify current habits that lead to over-treating low blood sugars, and create simple guidelines for treating lows without overeating.

Habits that Lead to Over-treating Low Blood Sugars:

- Using low blood sugars as an excuse to eat all of the foods you usually think of as "off-limits" or "bad."
- Being unprepared to treat lows by having specific foods nearby, which leads to impulsively eating any food in sight or during meals.
- Telling yourself that it's okay to overeat, because this is normal during a low blood sugar, and everybody does it.

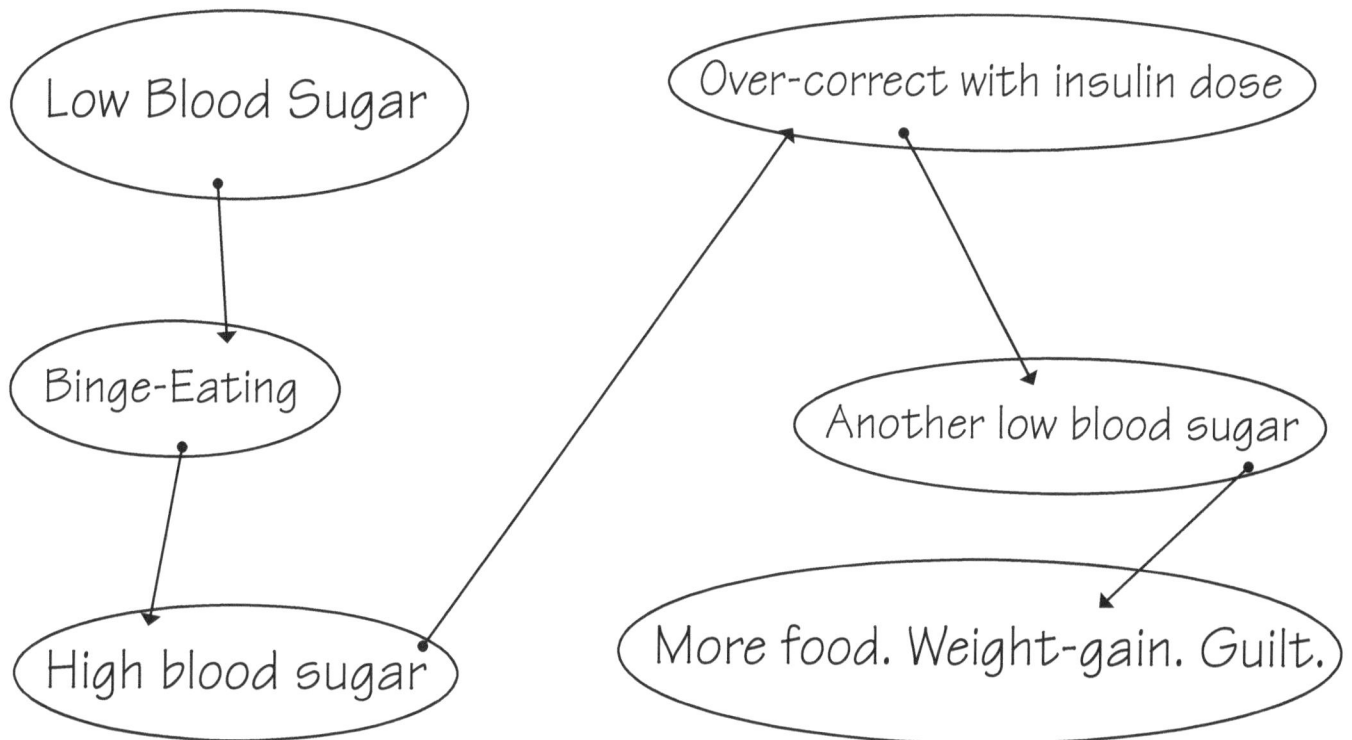

Low Blood Sugar → Binge-Eating → High blood sugar → Over-correct with insulin dose → Another low blood sugar → More food. Weight-gain. Guilt.

Gaining Weight from Over-treating Lows

Let's take a look at how many extra calories can be consumed from over-treating only one low blood sugar a week in these estimates:

Average low blood sugar binge
= 500 calories / low blood sugar

One 500 calorie binge per week
= 2,000 calories/month
= 24,000 calories/year

Recommended treatment for lows:
15 grams of carbohydrates = 60 calories

If we know that losing one pound of body fat requires that we burn or subtract 3,500 calories from our week, you can see how an extra 24,000 calories a year will interfere with your ability to lose weight.

Those extra 24,000 calories can lead to gaining approximately 7 pounds of body fat in one year.

Taking control over this area of your life is crucial for many reasons: blood sugar control, overall energy levels, happiness, and last but not least, managing your weight.

New Guidelines to Prevent Over-treating Your Lows:

- Foods you love (like ice cream, etc.) will be included in your nutrition plan and eaten when your blood sugar is in a safe range, and you can enjoy the meal. The foods you love will not be used to treat low blood sugars.

- Whenever possible, you will keep sources of carbohydrates for your low blood sugars nearby. These foods will be things you don't mind eating, but that you don't necessarily love. If you have a low right before a meal, you will use these foods to treat your low, so you can enjoy your meal without overeating.

- You will work to create a new habit in your thinking during a low: "My brain only needs _____ grams of carbohydrate in this moment. I need to be patient and give my brain time to catch up with my blood sugar. I will not abuse my body with food during this low."

The motivation to put these guidelines into action will come from acknowledging the consequences of your current habits. Consider how the stress from your current habit of over-treating your low blood sugars truly impacts every different area of your life: love, friendships, family, work, spirituality, physical health, and emotional health. Ask yourself, "How does my method of treating low blood sugars impact the people in my life who care about me?"

The moment you decide to take responsibility for the amount of food you put in your mouth during a low is the same moment you decide to put these guidelines into action and take control of this part of your life. Let's work on the details of **your** guidelines:

My Plan for Treating Lows

Personally, I can't stand the idea of going low, then high, then low again after over-correcting the high, and gaining weight from all those extra calories and extra insulin doses.

In order to prevent this roller-coaster in my own life with diabetes, I've created a plan for success:

By using foods I would probably never eat unless I was having a low blood sugar. The foods I choose are foods I don't dislike, but I don't really enjoy eating either. Juice of any kind, dried mangoes, gummy fruit snacks, glucose tabs, and bananas

I know that I would never over-indulge on any of these foods, no matter how much my brain might irrationally beg for more.

With these foods, I will consume only what I logically know I need, then I'll sit patiently and wait.

I keep these foods near my bed, in my car, under my desk at work, and in the kitchen. When I travel, I bring these foods with me to treat any lows.

My goal is to always be prepared

What foods do you use to treat low blood sugars that you abuse and overeat?

_____

_____

_____

_____

_____

_____

What foods can you use for lows that you will not be tempted to abuse and overeat?

_____

_____

_____

_____

_____

_____

Where will you store/place the foods listed above in order to be prepared for your lows?

_____

_____

_____

_____

_____

_____

While treating your low blood sugar, remind yourself repeatedly, **"I choose** how much food **I give myself."**

4 Using Food to Hide Your Emotions

Emotional eating looks different in every person's life. While sobbing into a carton of ice cream might be the stereotype you see on television, true emotional eating can be as subtle as sitting quietly on the couch after a long day at work, using a box of crackers and block of cheese as your tool for trying to unwind and relax.

Other days, emotional eating can take on a much more destructive nature.

Food can become a tool for self-punishment. It can become something you purposefully hurt yourself with while trying to show the world just how angry you are or how much you're hurting.

Food can become something you use for momentary comfort during an emotion or situation in your life that feels too immense, overwhelming, or scary to face on your own. Food becomes a tool to hide from or cover up anything.

In this chapter, we are going to look at four common situations in your life and your emotions that you may be using food to cover, ignore, or hide from. These common situations inevitably lead to a habit of overeating.

Before you read this chapter, here are a couple questions about your relationship with food for you to consider:

- Is your current relationship with food having an immensely negative impact on many different areas and relationships in your life?

- Are you ready to face this part of yourself and change your relationship with food?

If you're ready, then let's dig deeper:

The Disease You Didn't Ask For, That Won't Go Away

The first aspect of living with diabetes that may be influencing the way you treat your body with food is simply anger. Anger that your body has been diagnosed with a disease that requires constant attention, constant work, and there are no vacations. And that's putting it lightly. It impacts every part of your life.

Whether you're aware of this emotional burden on a regular basis, or you think about it rarely, or from time to time, the inevitable truth is that living with diabetes absolutely sucks.

Yes. I said it. Living with this disease sucks. Whether you are totally on top of your diabetes and it's a major priority in your life that has brought many positives with it, or you're struggling to take care of yourself, living with diabetes sucks.

You can't make this burden go away. But how you handle that burden and the emotions that come with it is up to you. Too often, you don't have a way to express just how angry you are about having to live with this disease. But now, it's time.

Are you abusing your body with food because you are angry at diabetes?

Are you angry that you have to live with this disease?

Wasting My Energy

Almost every day, I used to waste energy on small moments of road rage while driving. It's one of my worst habits, and I've been working hard to change it.

But it's simply that: a habit. Despite how much I dislike it, I am absolutely choosing to put my energy there. Choosing to waste my energy getting angry at people who sit at a traffic light for 10 seconds after its turned green.

Today, I remind myself it isn't worth my energy.

Living with diabetes, it would be easy to wake up every morning filled with resentment because I am a human pincushion, counting carbs every day and trying to do something for my body that it should do on its own.

I could spend my entire life wishing I didn't have diabetes, and hating the world for the fact that I do. To me, that is not worth my energy. It is a waste, just like those brief moments of road rage. Instead, I choose to put my energy towards accepting my life with diabetes, every single day.

Identifying Your Own Self-Worth and Self-Sabotage

Actions speak louder than words, right? If you genuinely believe that you and your body are worth kindness, compassion, and respect, the way you actually feed your body reveals the truth. The same can be said for how you exercise your body, the relationships you create in your life, and the thoughts you put in your own head about who you are and what you're worth.

Food is simply one way we reveal our beliefs of our own self-worth. Quite often, if you are disrespecting your body with food, you may also be allowing other people to disrespect you in your relationships. Also, you may be someone who puts everyone else's needs before your own, so you feel like you don't have time to exercise.

Do you truly believe you deserve to be healthy and happy?

The true answer to this question is crucial. As soon as you decide that you deserve good things in your life, you will begin to see the many habits or people in your life that are causing you more harm than good.

Deciding to treat your body with kindness means moderation, even if it's ice cream. It also means that you make time for yourself a priority, and make time for exercise. A person who decides they deserve to be happy doesn't have room in their life for people who continue to hurt them either emotionally or physically.

When you realize and believe your own personal worth, you will know **you** absolutely deserve health, happiness, and kindness in all things.

Abby Bayer's Story

"For most of my life, the extra aspects of diabetes played a secondary role. I checked my blood sugars and took my insulin, but exercise and healthy food wasn't a priority.

I only exercised if I had nothing better to do or had recently binged on junk food. I made excuses to not buy healthier foods: It's expensive. I can't cook, so it'll just go bad. I don't even like broccoli.

Now exercise is my plan after work, and I turn down less healthy alternatives on workout days. I go straight for the produce section of a grocery store first so that my basket is filled by the time I get to junk food.

Making these small changes doesn't automatically make my blood sugars perfect, but they have made me a much healthier and happier person.

This change didn't happen overnight, and my habits are still evolving, but instead of feeling guilty over my choices, I genuinely feel very proud of myself."

Rebelling Against the Rules: "You Can't Eat That"

"Diabetics cannot eat bread, pasta, candy and cookies." I'm sure you've heard, read, and been lectured about this many times in your life with diabetes. While you may think that putting this in your head regularly will help you abstain from these foods, it's more likely giving food much more power over you.

Ultimately, you can eat whatever you would like to eat. You're the one who picks it up and puts in your mouth. You have the final decision.

To believe that you cannot eat something is your choice, but the impact it leaves in your own mind might inevitably cause you to see that food as a way to fight back. It becomes a way break free from the demands of diabetes, and as a way to tell your parents, doctors, loved ones and the disease that they cannot control you. Your life is your own.

Labeling a food as "forbidden" makes that food much more enticing. The moment you feel overwhelmingly controlled, frustrated, or trapped in other areas of your life or specifically within diabetes, you will be much more likely to use food as an attempt to show the world, or specific people, that no one can tell you how to live your life.

Imagine if all food was available to you. Imagine if there were no rules, and ice cream was no longer any more desirable than carrots and hummus. Imagine if you simply decided: I can eat whatever I want. It is ultimately my own decision.

Suddenly, food will not resemble power or control. Instead, it's just food.

Jenny Smith's Story

"As someone who has lived with diabetes for over 24 years and also works as a Certified Diabetes Educator and Registered Dietitian, I absolutely do feel there is an overemphasis on the one thing in life that we cannot live without: food.

Regardless of diabetes, we all need food.

We need to eat! In appointments with doctors and diabetes educators, we focus so much on the negative consequences of food, instead of the many good things that food can give us, like fuel.

I try to focus on the other nutrients like protein and fat, while appreciating food for the good things it gives me. It helps me tremendously to keep that focus in mind while I'm at the grocery store.

In my own life with diabetes, I live an 80/20 plan. 80 percent of the time, I eat to fuel my life, 20 percent of the time, I eat because I choose to feed my desire for a treat—whatever that may be at the time!"

Unhappiness & Stress Over Things You Can't Change

Sometimes, there are parts of your life completely unrelated to food or diabetes that continue to feel incomplete. Things like friendship, love, career, body image, and overall happiness. You are human. We all need and want friendship, love, and happiness.

When you don't have one of these things in your life, food can become a quick and easy...well, not a substitute, but a **distraction**. Macaroni and cheese cannot replace love, and it never will. Eating too much of it, late at night, does not make your desire to find love or friendship go away. It is simply a way to ignore your feelings, needs, wants, and even insecurities.

Instead of trying to hide the fact that you feel loneliness and crave something like love, could you try to acknowledge it? Could you actually pause in the moment when you would usually reach for food, and say out loud, **"What I really want is love, not food."**

Write it down. Repeat it. **Acknowledge the truth.** While you certainly can't just walk out the door and find love, the first step to finding love, or whatever it is that you need or want in your life, is to acknowledge it, admit to it, and face it.

If you are using food to cover, hide, or distract yourself from emotions over a certain part of your life, those emotions or that situation will never evolve. They will continue to be hidden, covered with calories.

No matter what the unhappiness stems from, food isn't your solution. Uncover the truth and dig for the courage to turn toward it.

Mike Lawson's Story

"I love pancakes. After my diabetes diagnosis, I thought that I'd never enjoy pancakes again. Pancakes, which had once brought me joy, were now something on my plate that filled my head with thoughts.

Should I be eating this? I shouldn't be eating this. What's this going to do to my blood sugar later? I'm gonna regret this.

Even if I still decided to eat the pancakes, I wouldn't enjoy them because of everything going on in my head and the guilt that inevitably follows the meal. Eventually, I started learning how to correctly bolus for pancakes, through trial and error, and now I can predict what they will do to my blood sugar.

Today, when my blood sugar is high after eating pancakes, I knew I needed more insulin next time. It took a few years, but I've come to realize that with proper planning, I can have my pancakes and eat them too."

What is the first step to facing these emotions?

Changing the way you handle these emotions or situations in your life isn't going to happen overnight. And that's okay.

The first step is to simply face the truth. On your own, you have probably tried in the past to change your emotional eating by making new rules around food. Doing this doesn't actually address your emotions because it's simply another distraction. It doesn't actually give you what you need in order to change or cope with these parts of your life.

Instead of food, what do you actually need in this moment?

Facing this requires courage. The emotions or situation you're struggling with are not simple. To face those emotions is not easy. And that's okay. Remind yourself: this isn't supposed to be easy.

Whether it's something like anger over diabetes, pain from an unhealthy relationship, loneliness while struggling to find love, or an overwhelming pile of responsibilities in your lap, expressing how you truly feel by speaking the words aloud and even writing them down, is essential. Let it out.

If you have to cry for three days in order to get it all out, then cry. If you have to seek the help of a counselor to escape that relationship, then do it. If you have to ask your partner for help with all of those responsibilities, then ask. Again, it's time to dig for the courage to face this part of your life.

Ann Bartlett's Story

"My relationship with food is the mirror image of where I am with myself, and it is intensified and magnified by my life with diabetes.

In the course of a lifetime, that relationship is in constant change. I remember my teens being about fitting in, so I ate everything. There were no limits, no untouchables.

My twenties were about self-discovery and casting out inner demons. It was a time of purge and cleansing, physically and emotionally.

It was my choice to follow a very strict vegetarian diet, which lead into a very strict macrobiotic diet. This reflected how deeply I was trying to understand myself around food.

In my 40s, I found better balance while my life opened up into more strenuous tasks, higher stress, and physical needs that come with aging.

Today, food is about nutrition, but more importantly, my choices reflect the enjoyment of being confident and comfortable in who I am."

WORKSHEET #3 Expressing Your Emotions

Create a list of any of the emotions or situations of your life that can trigger you to overeat.

_____
_____
_____
_____
_____
_____
_____

Does overeating food make you feel better? If not, what does the food do for you?

_____
_____
_____
_____
_____
_____
_____

Are you purposefully hurting or punishing yourself with food? If yes, can you express why?

_____
_____
_____
_____
_____
_____
_____

How have you tried to change this part of your life that *has not* worked for you?

_____

_____

_____

_____

_____

_____

What have you *not tried yet* in order to change this part of your life?

_____

_____

_____

_____

_____

_____

Do you truly believe that you deserve happiness and health?

_____

_____

_____

_____

_____

_____

When you feel the urge to eat because of an emotion, **ask yourself**, "Instead of food, what do **I truly need** in this moment?"

⑤ A Positive Relationship with Food

How many times have you tried to change your relationship with food in the same way over and over, even though it doesn't ever truly help you?

This time, let's try something totally different.

In this chapter, I am going to ask you to let go of every rule around food you've read in a magazine, and to forget every lecture you've heard from someone telling you what to eat, and what not to eat.

I'm going to ask you to take down the walls and barriers and blockades you've designed inside your head about ice cream, or pizza, or potato chips...that have made those foods so powerfully forbidden, off-limits, and even more enticing.

I'm going to ask you to trust me, and try something you've never tried before. In this chapter we're going to design your new relationship with food.

Your new relationship with food will be based on healthy logic, with the understanding that you are human, you have a life that doesn't always fit a perfect schedule, and eating "perfectly" during every day of your entire life isn't actually a realistic or achievable goal.

Your New Guidelines include:
• Effective "rules" around food that will leave you feeling empowered in your choices.

• How to feed your body for proper energy levels, and give your metabolism the structure it needs to healthfully burn calories and fat.

• Creating a plan to include the treats you love in your overall relationship with food.

Okay, are you ready? Let's go.

Effective "Rules" for Your Positive Relationship with Food

- Fat, protein, and carbohydrates can all be part of my diet.
- I will eat when my body is hungry, even late at night.
- I can, if I choose to, eat any type of food that I want to eat.
- I will expect "imperfections" in my eating habits.
- I will feed my body regularly throughout the day.
- I will create a plan to include treats in my daily or weekly diet.
- Eating any sweets, treats, or junk food that I love is really okay.
- I will aim to give my body 80 to 90 percent healthy foods.
- I can enjoy treats, and I will enjoy them in moderation.
- All food is just food.

The guidelines you create and adapt to your life are meant to give you the freedom to make choices, rather than feel trapped around ideas of what you "should" or "shouldn't" eat. Your guidelines are also designed with the understanding that you are not perfect, and no one expects you to eat perfectly. Instead, we'll anticipate and plan for "less-than-perfect" foods, like the foods you love that you usually turn to when you binge. Your new guidelines make those foods acceptable, and part of your life, eventually making them useless for emotional needs.

In your new guidelines, there is no such thing as a "bad" food, because all food is just food. For some of you, cheese in moderation is part of a balanced nutrition plan. For others, cheese isn't appealing. If you love cheese, including it in moderation while looking at your entire day's nutrition can be part of your positive relationship with food. What does a balanced day of nutrition look like? Let's take a look:

Imperfect Diet = Balanced Mind

If someone told me I could never eat ice cream again, I know I would only want more ice cream. Instead, I almost always keep ice cream in my freezer. And I don't skimp with the light, low-fat stuff, either. This is **real** ice cream.

Do I overeat or abuse this ice cream? No, because it's always there. It's not forbidden, and therefore, not a big deal.

On nights when I know I want to eat ice cream, I cut back on my carbohydrate intake at dinner. If I know I'd rather eat rice, or several ears of corn

then I skip ice cream for that day, which allows me to keep within my personal goal for how many carbohydrates I consume in one day.

Is it possible that you might overeat that food you love when you first introduce it into your home and regular nutrition again?

Yes; however, if you continue to focus on how that food fits into your entire day of nutrition, and make room for its calories, it will no longer be a food you desperately abuse. Instead, it will become something you enjoy in moderation.

Eating to Fuel Your Metabolism

Imagine your doctor or dietitian has instructed you to eat 1,800 calories a day. If you eat two meals, of 900 calories each, your body is going to get an incredible amount of calories all at once. Some of it will be used for energy, the rest will be stored as fat.

Instead, by dividing your daily 1,800 calories into approximately four or five meals a day, you will be consuming 400 calories (give or take 50 to 100) per meal. Spread those four to five meals apart by three to four hours, and you will now be eating in a way that gives your metabolism a reason to burn calories more quickly during the entire day. You'll be eating only enough calories in one sitting so that your body won't be storing nearly as much food as body fat. **See example below.**

Below you'll also find that the day ends with 300 calories of ice cream, and yet the whole day's carbohydrate intake is still less than 100, which includes the low-glycemic carbohydrates from vegetables.

This nutrition sample reveals how you can still include sweets and treats in your life while keeping within the guidelines of a low-to-moderate carbohydrate plan (which is recommended for diabetes management and general weight loss). Even if you followed this outline of eating only five days a week, while consuming 200 grams of carbohydrates on Saturday and Sunday, you will reap the benefits.

Eating perfectly every single day is not the goal, mostly because it's not possible for most of us. Instead, you can focus on creating balance during five days of your week, including your treats, while fueling your metabolism and controlling your cravings.

A Day's Worth of Calories

This is a sample 1,800 calorie nutrition plan with five meals, spread evenly throughout the day, for a person who is following a low-to-moderate carbohydrate lifestyle. Calorie counts are an approximation from CalorieKing.com.

Breakfast: 1 egg + 3/4 cup egg whites, 4 slices of turkey bacon = approx. 300 calories

Lunch: mixed greens, 6 oz. sliced turkey, 2 tbsp. olive oil and vinegar, 1 slice swiss cheese, green peppers, and cucumbers – approx. 450 calories

Snack: 1 cup baby carrots, 1/4 cup hummus, 1 medium banana = approx. 350 calories

Dinner: 1 baked chicken breast without skin, 1 cup steamed broccoli and 1/2 cup steamed onions = approx. 375 calories

Snack: 1 - 1.5 cups ice cream = approx. 300 calories (varies greatly by brand)

Total calories: 1,775 calories
Total carbohydrates: 95 grams

Making Healthy Choices Around the Foods You Really Love

From this moment on, you are **allowed** to eat ice cream, potato chips, pizza, popcorn, and candy. When you eat those foods, there is no guilt or shame associated with that meal because you aren't doing anything wrong.

Does this sound absolutely crazy to you? Are you thinking, "Oh my goodness, I can't let myself eat those foods! I'll eat the whole carton or the whole bag or the whole box of pizza!"

Maybe. It's possible that you'll overdo it during the first day, or even the first week. That's okay, actually. Get it out of your system, and you will find yourself at the point where you don't want to gorge yourself with food all day. In fact, it doesn't feel good, especially when it's no longer food you had previously deemed "forbidden."

Ask yourself if trying to limit or restrain yourself from foods you love and crave has actually helped you want them less, or prevented you from binging on these foods during an emotional day or in response to feeling out of control? Chances are that the deprivation doesn't help.

Let's try something different: for some of you, including a treat once a day (yes, every day) is the best place to start. For others, every other day, or only on Saturday and Sunday is the right amount. You choose. Think about the food you love and how you'd like to include it in your life with self-respect and thoughtful purpose. Whether it's a special cheese with pepperoni on crackers, potato chips, or jelly beans, it's your choice.

Mari Ruddy's Plant-Based Diet

"As an athlete, a two-time breast-cancer survivor, and a person with type 1 diabetes and celiac disease, my diet is very fine-tuned for my needs: No meat. No dairy. No gluten. Here's a sample day of what I eat:

Breakfast: 4 oz orange juice, 3 scrambled egg whites cooked in coconut oil, veggies (spinach, arugula, mushrooms, onions, turmeric), 1 slice Udi's gluten-free bread

Snack: 6 walnuts, ½ apple

Lunch: Steamed beets, ear of fresh corn steamed, 1 tomato, black beans with Daiya nondairy cheese melted

Snack: ½ apple, cauliflower, hummus, Zevia Natural Soda, root beer

Dinner: Gluten-free spaghetti with squash sauce and fresh spinach, salad with veggies, oil and vinegar , 3 gluten-free ginger snap cookies

Snack: Frozen blueberries with a non-dairy milk (rice or almond milk)"

Create a list of the foods you love that you have labeled as "bad" and "off-limits."

_____

_____

_____

_____

_____

_____

_____

Let's create a specific weekly plan for how often you will make room for these foods:

_____

_____

_____

_____

_____

_____

_____

How will you adjust your nutrition on the days you make room for treats?

_____

_____

_____

_____

_____

_____

Create a list of your new "rules" around food:

_____

_____

_____

_____

_____

_____

_____

_____

_____

_____

_____

_____

_____

_____

_____

_____

_____

_____

_____

_____

_____

_____

Create an outline for feeding your body every 3 to 4 hours, Monday to Friday:

_____

_____

_____

_____

_____

_____

_____

_____

_____

_____

_____

_____

_____

_____

_____

_____

_____

_____

_____

_____

_____

_____

Think about
the food you love
and how you'd like
to include that food
in your life with
self-respect and
thoughtful purpose.

⑥ Setting Yourself Up for Success

There is, unfortunately, no **one-size-fits-all** nutrition program that we can all agree to follow for ultimate health and a perfect body.

We all have different needs when it comes to the ideal nutritional outline. Things like activity level, weight loss goals, taste buds, diabetes needs, gluten allergies, lactose intolerance, or choices like veganism, and what truly fits into our lives makes our needs different than our friends'.

Developing your new relationship with food takes time. You will learn how to expect that you just might fall "off the wagon," and how to get back on that wagon quickly.

In this chapter, you'll learn how to acknowledge personal progress in your evolving relationship with food. Believe it or not, the hardest part of your progress might be actually giving yourself credit for making progress! In the past, when you've tried to assess your progress, you may have been rather hard on yourself. Actually, too hard on yourself. You may have demanded perfection, and forgotten that you're human, and it takes time to change something immense in your life.

Yes, some theories say it takes 30 days to create a new habit, but you're not simply changing an action in your life—you're studying yourself and learning about your relationship with food. If you spend the next five years continuously evolving the choices you make around food, consider **that** incredible progress.

Your relationship with food is always evolving. What works for you this year might not fit in your life next year. Remind yourself, it takes time, and you're making progress day by day.

Let's begin with what happens when we feel like we've taken a step back, skip over the part where we beat ourselves up for it, and learn how to get back on track:

Falling "Off the Wagon" & Getting Back On that Wagon Quickly

Chances are, you will **not** go your entire life without overeating or emotionally binging ever again, even if you've gone weeks or months without a relapse. The difference between any future binges and your binges of the past lies in your ability to pick yourself up, dust yourself off, and get back on track.

Whether you fall off the wagon for one evening or two whole weeks, don't linger there with guilt. The moment you choose to acknowledge what you're doing, and decide that you'd like to stop, is the moment you launch your personal "Pick-up Plan."

Your "Pick-up Plan" consists of 3 steps:

- Acknowledge what happened: Write down or share with a friend exactly what led you to use food as an emotional outlet. Be as specific and honest as you can. Get it out. Acknowledge the truth. Turn towards it.
- Immediately forgive yourself: There is no room in your plan for guilt, shame, or self-blame. Instead, you will quickly and truly forgive yourself for abusing food. Write it down. Look at yourself in the mirror and forgive yourself for being human.
- Focus on Your "Pick-Up Phrase": Your "Pick-up Phrase" is a short sentence that helps you re-focus on your personal goals for your health and your relationship with food. Example: "I will feed my body with compassion and respect."

You will design your own "Pick-Up Plan" in this chapter's worksheet.

George Simmons' Story

"My love for food has always been a problem. As a kid I would eat when I was hungry, when others were eating, when I was bored, and whenever anything was in reach!

Those bad habits took a long time to break.

Something I read a few years back really changed the way I think about food. It basically asked, "Why jeopardize your entire body to please your taste buds?"

That really shook my foundation.

Thinking of food as fuel first and not just for pleasure really changes your perspective.

Now I find foods that I know are good fuel first and then find different ways to enjoy them.

There is great pleasure in knowing the food you are eating is healthy and that you are doing a good thing for your body.

It took a long time to find what worked for me but as long as we keep trying to change our bad habits, we will eventually. Just never stop trying!"

Acknowledging Your Progress

Surprisingly, one of the hardest parts of changing your relationship with food is actually stepping back to notice all of the progress you've made.

In the past, you may have judged your progress by weighing yourself every day, or counting calories. Instead, let's take a few steps back in order to think about your actual thoughts around food. The conversation and decision process that takes place in your head is the change that comes long before a change on the scale.

Maybe the changes you've made have also come from addressing other parts of your life, or your diabetes. By digging for the courage to face those parts of your life, you are purposefully working to create changes in how you treat your body with food. Give yourself a serious pat on the back for take this step forward!

Perhaps your progress has been that you've gone from eating half the carton of ice cream every night, without actually enjoying it, to actually making yourself a bowl of ice cream, counting the carbohydrates, and enjoying every spoonful. That is progress!

Whether you create a list of your improvements week-by-week on a giant poster board in your bedroom, or you tell your best friend over the phone every now and then, it's important stop and look at the finer details of your personal evolution around food.

Remember, it's not about perfection. If you "make a mistake" in one or several parts of your day, that does not mean you've failed. You're human and constantly evolving. Be kind to yourself, and keep going.

Noticing Small Improvements

These are just a few of the seemingly small steps of progress that are incredibly significant:

• After you overeat due to emotion, stress, or boredom, you are able to acknowledge what happened honestly.

• When you realize you've overeaten or abused food, you are able to tell yourself, "Okay. That happened. Let's move on." No guilt.

• You are eating breakfast regularly!

• You are making thoughtful decisions around the food at work, parties, and holidays in order to maintain a balance.

• You are enjoying the food you eat, the healthy meals and the treats, too.

• You're eating small meals, often.

• Frequently, you ask yourself, "Am I actually hungry... or do I want food for an entirely different reason?"

In your own words, outline the 3 steps of your Pick-up Plan:

_____

_____

_____

_____

_____

_____

_____

_____

_____

_____

_____

_____

_____

How do you plan to track your own progress? Brainstorm a few ideas here:

_____

_____

_____

_____

_____

_____

_____

_____

_____

_____

_____

You don't have to
be perfect.
You are **human**.
You will make
mistakes.
Pick yourself up
and get back
on track.

7 You Are Living in Progress

"It would be so much easier if we didn't have to eat in order to survive. It makes everything so much more complicated." My friend Scott Johnson said this with frustration about food and diabetes.

His statement is poignant, and true. How wonderful would it be if eating was as unessential to our life as putting polish on our fingernails or painting flames on the back of our car?

Instead, food is a crucial part of every living thing's life. Weeds, flowers, bumblebees, fish, lions, babies, teenagers, and adults. You all need food. Some creatures and people desperately struggle to find enough food, while others struggle to keep themselves from eating too much.

No human, creature, or plant is free from having to think about the food in their life. Too much or too little for any of us has consequences. No one gets to live around food without those consequences. Adding diabetes to that equation is simply another challenge on our plates.

There is no shortcut. The world has tried to create pills, surgery, and diets around food to change the challenge, and some of those things might help, but in the end it will still come down to the choices we make, the food we put in our own mouths, and how we create our own relationship with food.

Whether we choose to call it willpower, knowledge, self-respect, or a personal life philosophy, we are in charge of how we feed our bodies, and how we respect or disrespect ourselves around food.

You don't have to be perfect. In fact, you should anticipate that you won't and can't be perfect. Gradual improvement is the goal. Allow yourself the freedom to make mistakes. And decide that you'll never give up. Never give up.

Your relationship with food is in constant progress. **Give yourself** the freedom to learn, make mistakes, and **gradually evolve.**

* Resources & Support

Professional Coaching, Therapy & Diabetes Education
• Wellness & Diabetes Coaching • Living-in-Progress.com • Ginger Vieira CHC, CPT
• Go-with-Your-Gut Coaching • Go-With-Your-Gut.com • Ilise Ratner MA, CHC
• Behavioral Diabetes Inst. • BehavioralDiabetesInstitute.org • William Polonsky PhD, CDE
• Integrated Diabetes Services • IntegratedDiabetes.com • Gary Scheiner MS, CDE
• Team WILD Athletics • TeamWILDathletics.com • Mari Ruddy & Coaches
• Art Therapy • LeeAnnThill.com • Lee Ann Thill MA, ATR-BC, LPC

Books for Continued Learning
• Food Rules - An Eater's Manual - Michael Pollan
• The Ultramind Solution - Mark Hyman MD
• The Blood Sugar Solution - Mark Hyman MD
• Your Diabetes Science Experiment - Ginger Vieira CHC, CPT
• The Eat-Clean Diet - Tosca Reno
• The Diabetes Miracle - Diane Kress RD, CDE
• Integrative Nutrition - Joshua Rosenthal MScED
• Think Like A Pancreas - Gary Scheiner MS, CDE
• Diabetes Meal Planning Made Easy - Hope Warshaw RD, CDE

Diabetes Websites and Blogs
• YouTube.com/MrMikeLawson - Mike Lawson
• ScottsDiabetes.com - Scott Johnson
• DiabetesSocMed.com - Cherise Shockley
• Ninjabetic.com - George Simmons
• SixUntilMe.com - Abby Bayer
• BodyInBalanceCenter.com - Ann Bartlett
• DiabetesAdvocates.org
• DiabetesDaily.com
• YouCanDoThisProject.com
• TuDiabetes.org
• MyGlu.org

Thank you

This book is the result of many amazing friends, colleagues, and family. My mother, Marlita, and sister, Alyssa, will always be my greatest editors. My friends Tara, Dana, Jen, and Beth are wonderful readers, reviewers and supporters. I'm lucky to call you my friends!

Mike Lawson, Scott Johnson, Cherise Shockley, George Simmons, Abby Bayer, Ann Bartlett, Jenny Smith, Mari Ruddy, David Edelman, and Dr. Polonksy: thank you for your time, energy, and support in the creation of this book! You are brilliant advocates, and I appreciate your support.

Chris Valites and Jess Piccirilli, I look forward to working with both of you again. Chris, I so appreciate your commitment to making your work turn out just right! Jess, you saved the day.

To the students at Champlain's Publishing Initiative, I am so grateful for your energy and passion as you build your already impressive skills in writing and publishing. Thank you all for dedicating your time to this project.

Tim Brookes! I continue to learn from you, many years after graduation. I'd say you're worth every cent of college tuition. Thank you for everything you continue to do.

To the Diabetes Online Community, you are everywhere and you are incredible. Thank you for everything you do. Living with this disease is no easy feat, and you're doing it. Every day.

Never give up.

> With love and gratitude,
> Ginger

About The Champlain College Publishing Initiative

The Champlain College Publishing Initiative has been created in order to engage as many of our students as possible in the field of publishing, whether as writers, editors, designers, artists, marketers, publicists, accountants, or web designers, to give them a supervised educational experience that is creative, demanding, and applicable to the world they meet when they graduate.

Our mission is to play an active part in the great experiment that is contemporary publishing.

Visit us at www.ChamplainCollegePublishing.com

www.ingramcontent.com/pod-product-compliance
Lightning Source LLC
Chambersburg PA
CBHW051346290326
41933CB00042B/3302

www.ingramcontent.com/pod-product-compliance
Lightning Source LLC
Chambersburg PA
CBHW051350290326
41933CB00042B/3355